Patient	Location
Concerns	Family
Notes	

Patient	Location
Concerns	Family

Notes

Patient	Location
Concerns	Family

Notes

Patient	Location
Concerns	Family

Notes

Patient	Location
Concerns	Family
Notes	

Patient	Location
Concerns	Family

Notes

Patient	Location
Concerns	Family

Notes

Patient	*Location*
Concerns	*Family*

Notes

Patient	Location
Concerns	Family

Notes

Patient	Location
Concerns	Family

Notes

Patient	Location
Concerns	Family

Notes	

Patient	Location
Concerns	Family

Notes

Patient	Location
Concerns	Family

Notes

Patient	Location
Concerns	Family

Notes

Patient	Location
Concerns	Family

Notes	

Patient	Location
Concerns	Family

Notes

Patient	Location
Concerns	Family

Notes

Patient	Location
Concerns	Family

Notes

Patient	Location
Concerns	Family

Notes

Patient	*Location*
Concerns	*Family*

Notes

Patient	Location
Concerns	Family

Notes

Patient	Location
Concerns	Family

Notes

Patient	Location
Concerns	Family

Notes

Patient	Location
Concerns	Family

Notes

Patient	Location
Concerns	Family

Notes

Patient	Location
Concerns	Family
Notes	

Patient	Location
Concerns	Family

Notes

Patient	Location
Concerns	Family

Notes

Patient	Location
Concerns	Family

Notes

Patient	Location
Concerns	Family

Notes

Patient	Location
Concerns	Family

Notes

Patient	Location
Concerns	Family

Notes

Patient	Location
Concerns	Family

Notes

Patient	Location
Concerns	Family

Notes

Patient	Location
Concerns	Family

Notes

Patient	*Location*
Concerns	*Family*

Notes

Patient	Location
Concerns	Family

Notes

Patient	Location
Concerns	Family

Notes

Patient	Location
Concerns	Family

Notes

Patient	Location
Concerns	Family

Notes

Patient	Location
Concerns	Family

Notes

Patient	Location
Concerns	Family

Notes

Patient	Location
Concerns	Family

Notes

Patient	Location
Concerns	Family

Notes

Patient	Location
Concerns	Family

Notes

Patient	Location
Concerns	Family

Notes

Patient	Location
Concerns	Family

Notes

Patient	Location
Concerns	Family

Notes

Patient	Location
Concerns	Family

Notes

Patient	Location
Concerns	Family

Notes

Patient	Location
Concerns	Family

Notes

Patient	Location
Concerns	Family

Notes

Patient	Location
Concerns	Family

Notes

Patient	Location
Concerns	Family

Notes

Patient	Location
Concerns	Family

Notes	

Patient	Location
Concerns	Family

Notes

Patient	Location
Concerns	Family

Notes

Patient	Location
Concerns	Family

Notes

Patient	Location
Concerns	Family

Notes

Patient	Location
Concerns	Family
Notes	

Patient	Location
Concerns	Family

Notes

Patient	Location
Concerns	Family

Notes

Patient	Location
Concerns	Family

Notes

Patient	Location
Concerns	Family

Notes

Patient	Location
Concerns	Family

Notes

Patient	Location
Concerns	Family

Notes

Patient	Location
Concerns	Family

Notes

Patient	Location
Concerns	Family

Notes

Patient	Location
Concerns	Family

Notes

Patient	Location
Concerns	Family
Notes	

Patient	Location
Concerns	Family
Notes	

Patient	Location
Concerns	Family

Notes

Patient	Location
Concerns	Family

Notes

Patient	Location
Concerns	Family

Notes

Patient	Location
Concerns	Family

Notes

Patient	Location
Concerns	Family

Notes

Patient	Location
Concerns	Family

Notes

Patient	Location
Concerns	Family

Notes

Patient	Location
Concerns	Family

Notes

Patient	Location
Concerns	Family

Notes

Patient	Location
Concerns	Family

Notes

Patient	Location
Concerns	Family
Notes	

Patient	Location
Concerns	Family

Notes

Patient	Location
Concerns	Family

Notes

Patient	Location
Concerns	Family

Notes

Patient	Location
Concerns	Family

Notes

Patient	Location
Concerns	Family

Notes

Patient	Location
Concerns	Family

Notes

Patient	Location
Concerns	Family

Notes

Patient	Location
Concerns	Family
Notes	

Patient	Location
Concerns	Family

Notes

Patient	Location
Concerns	Family

Notes

Patient	Location
Concerns	Family

Notes

Patient	Location
Concerns	Family

Notes

Patient	Location
Concerns	Family

Notes

Patient	Location
Concerns	Family

Notes

Patient	Location
Concerns	Family
Notes	

Patient	Location
Concerns	Family

Notes

Patient	Location
Concerns	Family

Notes

Patient	Location
Concerns	Family

Notes

Patient	Location
Concerns	Family

Notes

Patient	Location
Concerns	Family

Notes

Patient	Location
Concerns	Family

Notes

Patient	Location
Concerns	Family

Notes

Patient	Location
Concerns	Family

Notes

Patient	Location
Concerns	Family

Notes

Patient	Location
Concerns	Family

Notes

Patient	Location
Concerns	Family

Notes

Patient	Location
Concerns	Family

Notes

Patient	Location
Concerns	Family

Notes

Patient	Location
Concerns	Family

Notes

Patient	Location
Concerns	Family

Notes

Patient	Location
Concerns	Family

Notes

Patient	Location
Concerns	Family

Notes

Patient	Location
Concerns	Family

Notes

Patient	Location
Concerns	Family

Notes

Patient	Location
Concerns	Family

Notes

Patient	*Location*
Concerns	*Family*

Notes

Patient	Location
Concerns	Family

Notes

www.ingramcontent.com/pod-product-compliance
Lightning Source LLC
Chambersburg PA
CBHW030711220526
45463CB00005B/1997